Juicing for Sexual Health

The Ultimate Beginners' Smoothie Guide for increasing Libido, boost Sex Drive and last longer in Bed without Pills

Kevin Mary Neo

Table of Contents

Introduction

Dwindling libidos is actually a resultant after-effect of emotional trauma, financial pressures, stress at work, insufficient enthusiasm, monotony, unhealthy lifestyle and diet plan, etc. Whatever the reason, there's a way to really get your groove again and satisfy your companion naturally without heavy reliance on performance enhancement drugs like Viagra

Sex is among the greatest pleasures on the planet, since it serves a number of purposes, from relaxation to pleasure and sometimes manipulation. In whatever case it might be, we all come with an inbuilt desire to enjoy and provide our partners the sexual satisfaction they crave, therefore the art of sex itself will not become an ordeal; a required evil.

Sadly, many couples are losing the sexual spark they once shared inside the bedroom, to an array of reasons which dwindling libidos worsened by unhealthy lifestyle choices defined as the major culprit.

This is actually the main purpose of this book. We will look into some typically common natural drink recipes, smoothies that boost sexual drive and libido in men and women.

Shall we begin.

Chapter 1

Sex Boosting Smoothie recipes and preparation

Ingredients

- ✓ 1/2 ripe banana
- ✓ 1/2 ripe avocado
- ✓ 1/2 hand filled with soaked almonds cups
- ✓ 1 tablespoon of coconut oil
- ✓ 1 teaspoon of raw chocolate powder
- ✓ 2 teaspoons of Maca
- ✓ 1 half teaspoon of Ashwagandha
- ✓ Pinch of cinnamon
- ✓ A little bit of honey

What else would you need?

- ✓ Blender or hand blender

How exactly to do it?

- ✓ Peel the banana
- ✓ Spoon the avocado out
- ✓ Pour everything right into a jar
- ✓ Blend everything together

✓ Decorate with cinnamon

Additional Tips

Drink each day for breakfast, or after your exercise with some protein powder added, or one hour before your sex date.

Variations welcome: Put your preferred fruit or boost with some berries.

Chocolate Peanut Butter Smoothie

This grounds chocolate is recognized as an aphrodisiac: It releases dopamine, the brain's pleasure chemical. This sexy smoothie also includes the amino acid L-arginine to transport healthy blood circulation to sex organs, as well as libido lifting vitamin D, B, and zinc.

✓ 1¼ c skim milk

✓ ¼ c plain Greek yogurt

✓ 1 Tbsp natural peanut butter

✓ 1 Tbsp cocoa powder

✓ 1 frozen banana

✓ Handful of ice

Blend until smooth and serve. Serves 1.

Banana Smoothie with Ginger

Juice the primary 3 ingredients properly, and put the banana. For banana, you should use blender since it will clog juicer extractor.

- ✓ Watermelon, enjoy 1 cup cubed with rind
- ✓ Fresh 5-10 cherries without the pits
- ✓ 1" clean ginger with your skin
- ✓ 1 banana.

Strawberry Vanilla Smoothie

The following can be an ideal afternoon smoothie. Blend all of the ingredient's in accurate measurements. Stop whenever you have a flavorful and superb textured smoothie inside your glass.

- ✓ 1 cup of strawberries (frozen)
- ✓ 1 tablespoon vanilla extract
- ✓ 1 cup almond milk (unsweetened).

Raspberries with Cinnamon

That is an ultimate penile enlargement smoothie. Position the ingredients one at a time, juice them until you find your desired smoothie.

- ✓ 1¼ cup raspberries (frozen)
- ✓ 1½ tablespoon hemp seeds
- ✓ 1½ cup of water
- ✓ ½ tablespoon cinnamon

Strawberry Stress Buster

Red may be the color of passion, so when it involves the red hue of strawberries, these ovary-shaped aphrodisiac fruits are thought to increase passion and promote healthy blood circulation to the brain and extremities. The bitterness in these berries also indicates their ability to activate the liver in removing hormones that the body no longer needs. By combining strawberries with magnesium-rich almond milk, the agitation and sleeplessness are combated while providing an ample dose of vitamin C. Adding vanilla into the mix brings awareness to the genitals, as this potent herb is known to cause urethral irritation.

Combine the next measurements of ingredients and blend until smooth to get a flavorful and beneficial afternoon pick-me-up.

- ✓ 1½ c unsweetened almond milk
- ✓ 1 c frozen strawberries
- ✓ 1 tsp vanilla extract.

Raspberry Zinger

Buying smoothie that's sure to really get your sexual juices flowing? Search no further than this raspberry zinger. Raspberries build blood and increase passion, while hemp seeds work to improve sex hormone production. The raspberry and hemp seed combination works to improve the metabolism of fat that promotes circulation, and cinnamon warms your body and increases libido.

Combine the next ingredients and blend until smooth for the best libido-boosting smoothie.

- ✓ 1½ Tbsp hemp hearts (shelled hemp seeds)
- ✓ 1¼ c frozen raspberries
- ✓ 1½ c water
- ✓ ½ tsp cinnamon

To maximize the consequences with the abundant treasures hidden in nature, light exercises ought to be added to obtain your information and retain your blood pumping.

Chapter 2

Smoothie Recipes for Increased Libido and Sexual Drive

Avocado Smoothies

Avocado-Smoothie-Recipe

They are saturated in folic acids, and so are an excellent source of vigor boost needed to keep things raunchy inside the bedroom. In addition, they contain healthy fats, Vitamin B and potassium; which function as a booster of male hormones necessary for virility in the bedroom.

Ingredients

- ✓ 2 large balls of avocado pears (seeds removed)
- ✓ ½ cup of frozen pineapples
- ✓ 1 cup of Almond milk
- ✓ 10 grams of ginger

Directions

- ✓ Place the seeded avocado within the blender
- ✓ Contribute the frozen pineapples
- ✓ Supply the ginger plus the Almond milk

✓ Blend everything together until smooth

✓ Pour in a glass and then add ice.

Watermelon Smoothies

Watermelon-Smoothie

This scarlet beauty is packed with Citrulline which aids the relaxation and dilation of arteries. Just about performing exactly the same functions as prescription medications targeted at treating erectile dysfunctions.

Ingredients

✓ 1 cup of watermelon with the seeds

✓ 1 little bit of apple (diced)

✓ 10 grams of ginger

✓ 1 cup of Almond milk or unsweetened yoghurt.

Directions

✓ Pour watermelon into the blender

✓ Put your apple and grated ginger

✓ Bring your milk or Yoghurt

✓ Blend everything together until smooth

✓ Pour right into a glass and serve with ice

✓ Pumpkins Seed Smoothies

Maca or Peruvian Ginseng

Maca or Peruvian Ginseng juice

This super fruit is native to the southern American and considered an *adaptogen*, at the top of the set of its immense benefits is increased testosterone as well as the tremendous boost it offers sex and fertility. *Increased intake of the black maca shows improved sperm production.*

Ingredients

- ✓ 1 tablespoon of dried maca powder.
- ✓ 1 cup of frozen Bananas.
- ✓ 1 or ½ cup of yoghurt or Almond milk.

Directions

- ✓ Pour your frozen bananas inside a blender.
- ✓ Add your yoghurt or almond milk to it.
- ✓ Then put a tablespoon of maca powder to the mixture.
- ✓ Blend until the mixture is smooth.

✓ Pour in a glass as well as your smoothie is ready.

Strawberry Stress Buster

Red may be the color of passion, so when it involves the red hue of strawberries, these ovary-shaped aphrodisiac fruits are thought to increase passion and promote healthy blood circulation to the mind and extremities. The bitterness in these berries also indicates their capability to activate the liver in removing hormones that the body no longer needs. By combining strawberries with magnesium-rich almond milk, the agitation and sleeplessness are combated while providing an ample dose of vitamin C. Adding vanilla into the mix brings awareness to the genitals, as this potent herb is known to cause *urethral irritation*.

Combine the next measurements of ingredients and blend until it is smooth for any flavorful and beneficial afternoon pick-me-up.

✓ 1½ c unsweetened almond milk
✓ 1 c frozen strawberries
✓ 1 tsp vanilla extract

Pomegranate Juice

Pomegranate-Juice-Nutrition-and-Benefits

Pomegranates contain powerful anti-oxidants and were first regarded as the *symbol of fertility*. According to Researchers from your Queen Margaret University, One glass of pomegranate increases testosterone levels, acting as an all-natural aphrodisiac.

The analysis also proves they contain certain compounds comparable to sex steroids found within humans; this explains the partnership between pomegranates and increased sexual stamina and desires

Ingredients

- ✓ 1 cup of seeded pomegranates.
- ✓ 20 grams of ginger.
- ✓ 1 medium Lemon (juiced).

Directions

- ✓ Pour the seeded pomegranates inside a blender.
- ✓ Bring your peeled and cut ginger.
- ✓ Add the juiced lemon and a cup of water.

✓ Blend the mixture until very smooth.

✓ Pour out into a glass and then add ice.

✓ Your smoothie is set to be consumed.

Chapter 3

Celery Smoothie

Celery-smoothie and drink

They may be laced with *vitamin E, niacin, potassium, and magnesium*. In addition, it contains arginine, an amino acid which performs the same work as a sex enhancement by aiding the expanding of arteries.

Ingredients

- ✓ 2 cups of celery leaves
- ✓ 1 green apple (diced)
- ✓ 1 lemon(juiced)
- ✓ Almond or unsweetened yoghurt

Directions

- ✓ Pour your properly washed celery into a blender
- ✓ Put your apples and juiced lemon
- ✓ Add your almond milk or yoghurt
- ✓ Blend until smooth
- ✓ Pour in a cup then add ice and it is done to be consumed

Goji Berry or Wolf Berry Smoothie

Wolf Berry Juice

These berries are native to Asia and also have high anti-oxidant properties. It's mostly prepared like a sexual tonic to *boost sexual drive and stamina*. Consumption of Goji berries has been thought to increase testosterone levels, Improve sexual abilities, increase sperm quality and movement. Researchers have suggested increased consumption of Goji as a wholesome alternative to prescription of medications for erectile dysfunctions like Viagra.

Ingredients

- ✓ 1 peeled Banana
- ✓ ½ cup of dried Goji berries (soaked for a handful of hours)
- ✓ 10 grams of ginger
- ✓ 1 cup of Almond milk

Directions

- ✓ Pour the diced into the blender
- ✓ Supply your softened goji berries

- ✓ Put your diced ginger and almond milk
- ✓ Blend until mixture is smooth
- ✓ Pour in a glass and Serve with Ice.

The libido-enhancing smoothie becomes set to be enjoyed together with your lover.

Pumpkins Seed Smoothie

These are heavily packed with *potassium, niacin, calcium, phosphorus, and zinc,* which really is a prerequisite for the production of healthy sperms while boosting testosterone levels. Also, they are heavily packed with libido enhancing vitamins like *Vitamin B, C, K, D, E.*

Ingredients

- ✓ 1 tablespoon of pumpkin seeds
- ✓ ½ cup of frozen pineapples
- ✓ ½ cup of frozen bananas
- ✓ 1 cup of unsweetened yoghurt.

Directions

- ✓ Pour your frozen pineapples inside a blender
- ✓ Put your bananas and pumpkin seeds

- ✓ Supply your yoghurt
- ✓ And blend everything together until smooth
- ✓ Pour in a glass and serve with ice.

Bananas Smoothie

Banana Smoothie and drink

Bananas are abundant with *potassium, magnesium, vitamin B1, vitamin A, Vitamin C, and Protein*; which are necessary for the improvement and production of sperms. In addition, it contains Bromelain, an enzyme in charge of increased libido and reversal of impotence in men.

Ingredients

- ✓ 2 mid-sized bananas peeled
- ✓ 10 grams of ginger
- ✓ 1 cup of Almond milk
- ✓ ½ cup of washed celery leaves

Directions

- ✓ Pour your diced bananas within a blender
- ✓ Add the celery leaves as well as your grated ginger
- ✓ Supply your almond milk to the mix

✓ And blend before the mixture is usually smooth
✓ Pour in a glass and then add ice as well as your smoothie is ready.

Beet root Smoothie

Beets continues to be used for years and praised as the best food for men, and it is abundant with *vitamin C and essential minerals like manganese and potassium.*

Frequent consumption of beetroots has immense benefits for health generally and libido specifically because they are highly concentrated with nitrates that get divided into nitric oxide. *Nitric oxide* generated by beetroots supports blood flow towards the penis, producing a stronger, fuller and sustained erection; giving the person a viagra-like effect, without medical effects of Viagra.

Ingredients

✓ mid-sized Beetroot
✓ 3 bits of Celery Stalks
✓ 1 medium Lemon juiced
✓ 20 grams of ginger

- ✓ 1 medium apple
- ✓ 1 cup of clean water

Directions

- ✓ Wash all of your vegetables with clean water and one tablespoon of vinegar
- ✓ Cut them into small pieces prepared to be blended
- ✓ Pour in a blender
- ✓ Blend until smooth
- ✓ Pour in a glass and add ice
- ✓ And Voila! your juice is set to be consumed.

Banana Booster

Two things one thinks of when it comes to bananas: smiles and undoubtedly penises. Bananas are aphrodisiac, providing long-term energy and stamina as well as stimulating the production of serotonin, which helps improve sleep and elevate mood. Adding chia seeds into the mix transforms this smoothie into an energy tonic that moistens yin energy *(feminine)*. Beyond these benefits, this dairy-free smoothie is jam-packed with the *feel-good chemical* **dopamine**, along with *zinc, magnesium and vitamin B6*, all shown to have effects on improving mood.

Blend the first three ingredients until smooth, bring the rest of the ingredients, blend and serve. This recipe serves one.

- ✓ ¼ c raw cashews
- ✓ 2 pitted dates
- ✓ 1¼ c water
- ✓ 1 frozen banana
- ✓ 1 Tbsp chia seeds
- ✓ Handful of ice

Carrots Smoothie

This orange beauty will not just leave your skin layer glowing, as well as your immunity high, but it additionally does wonders for sexual health.

Studies show that men who eat carrots at least 4 times weekly show a rise in sperm fertility and sexual prowess inside the bedroom.

Ingredients

- ✓ 1 cup of diced carrots
- ✓ 1 medium apple

- ✓ ½ cup of diced pineapples
- ✓ 10 grams of ginger

Direction

- ✓ Pour your diced or shredded carrots into the blender
- ✓ Put your diced apples and pineapples
- ✓ Put in a glass of water as well as your grated gingers
- ✓ Blend your ingredients together until smooth
- ✓ Pour in a glass and then add cubes of ice which are prepared to drink.

Chocolate Strawberry Banana Smoothie

Ingredients

- ✓ 1/2 frozen banana
- ✓ 1/4 cup strawberries, fresh or frozen
- ✓ 1/4 cup peaches, fresh or frozen
- ✓ 1 tablespoon raw pumpkin seeds
- ✓ 1 tablespoon chocolates (70-percent cocoa or even more)
- ✓ 1/2 cup chocolates almond milk
- ✓ 1/2 cup cool water
- ✓ 1/8 teaspoon ginger

Directions

Pour ingredients into a blender, blend until smooth, and revel in!

Chocolate Peanut Butter Smoothie

Cocoa beans have always been used to improve libido. This aphrodisiac was so potent that it had been actually prescribed by physicians in the 1800s as a reliable remedy for a minimal libido. Chocolate was known as *"food for the gods"* by the **Aztecs** due to its capability to release dopamine, which is the brain's pleasure chemical. With the combination of *peanut butter and banana,* this smoothie is usually filled up with *vitamin D and B, zinc and contains the amino acid L-arginine* which promotes healthy blood flow to sex organs.

Combine these ingredients and blend until it becomes smooth for an energizing smoothie which is able to maintain you up in more ways than one!

- ✓ 1¼ c skim milk
- ✓ ¼ c plain Greek yogurt
- ✓ 1 Tbsp natural peanut butter

- ✓ 1 Tbsp cocoa powder
- ✓ 1 frozen banana
- ✓ Handful of ice

Chapter 4

Super Sex boosting Foods

Avocado

Avocado-healthy and delicious aphrodisiacs

This rich and creamy fruit continues to be considered an aphrodisiac dating back to the Aztec time. Back then it had been because of its sensuous pear shape, and even though that shape still helps avocado look appealing, its high degrees of vitamin E is actually what it's known for. Vitamin E is thought to support one, and maintain youthful vigor and energy, as well as assist in lubrication.

Bananas

Bananas-healthy and delicious aphrodisiacs

Bananas are not just nice and delicious,they are also packed with vitamin B and potassium, which are two essential elements in the production of sex hormones. Bananas are also filled with chelating nutrients, which help your body absorb essential nutrients and so are therefore thought to raise the male libido.

Dark Chocolate

Dark Chocolate healthy and delicious aphrodisiacs

Another reason chocolate makes an ideal gift to your Valentine! Chocolate contains *L-arginine*, an amino acid that increases nitric oxide and promotes blood circulation to sexual organs for men and women. L-arginine may also assist in sensation and satisfaction. Additionally, chocolate also includes phenylethylamine and theobromine. The compound theobromine might help you feel activated and excited, and phenylethylamine helps improves moods by increasing serotonin levels.

Figs

Figs-Healthy and delicious aphrodisiacs

Figs have already been around for years and were Cleopatra's favorite fruit. The ancient Greeks associated them with love and fertility, and with justification! Figs are saturated in flavonoids and antioxidants, that may assist in sexual stamina.

Watermelon

Watermelon-healthy and delicious aphrodisiacs

This hydrating fruit contains citrulline, a plant nutrient recognized to benefit the cardiovascular and disease-fighting capability. *Citrulline* can be thought to work similarly to Viagra, for the reason that it relaxes arteries and improves blood circulation.

Honey

Honey is a healthy and delicious aphrodisiacs
Honey does a lot more than sweeten; it's also an excellent way to obtain boron, which includes been shown to greatly help stimulate estrogen production in women and testosterone production in men. Honey can be thought to increase nitric oxide levels, which may be the chemical released during arousal. No wonder it's a term of endearment!

Arugula

arugula-healthy and delicious aphrodisiacs
Arugula offers reportedly have been used as an aphrodisiac because of the initial century. Research shows that this trace minerals and antioxidants in dark, leafy greens are crucial for sexual health because they help

block environmental contaminants that may negatively affect our libidos.

Chili Peppers

Chili Peppers- healthy and delicious aphrodisiacs

Maintain things hot and spicy with this aphrodisiac. *Chili peppers* support the chemical capsaicin, which helps increase circulation, heart rate, induce sweating, and raise the sensitivity of nerve endings. Capsaicin can be an all-natural irritant, so it's recognized to result in a stinging, tingling sensation - adding a spark and sizzle to every kiss.

Pine Nuts

Pine nuts do a lot more than put in a zest to some dish, they are able to also reportedly assist with sexual stamina in men. That is because of the high zinc content, which protects against impotence and infertility.

Strawberries

Strawberries-Healthy and Delicious Aphrodisiacs

Strawberries dipped in chocolate will be the ultimate Valentine's Day treat! Maybe it is because strawberries are abundant with folic acid and vitamin C, which may help increase sperm fertility and improve sperm motility.

Pomegranates

Pomegranate-Aphrodisiacs.

The abundance of antioxidants in pomegranates give this fruit its aphrodisiac qualities. Antioxidants protect the liner of arteries, allowing more blood to course through them, which helps increase genital sensitivity.

Raw Chocolate

The entire world loves chocolate. There have been 3.97 million a lot of cocoa beans stated in 2008-2009. That's incredible there should be something to it that it's almost everyone's favorite treat, but magic is in the beans (that aren't sweet) not the sugar. Chocolate originates from cocoa beans. Raw cocoa was also termed the nourishment in the gods by the Aztecs. It's a superfood with tons of antioxidants and stimulating chemicals such as phenylethylamine which stimulates the sense of excitement and well-being. The Journal of Sexual Medicine published a study that found that women who enjoy a piece of chocolate on a daily basis have a more active sex life than those you don't.

Maca

Maca is really a trendy superfood from Peru. And it deserves to shine: It grows 4,100 m above sea level in the Andes. Maca may be the energizing and revitalizing superfood of the Incas, who revered it because of its aphrodisiac qualities and wide-ranging advantages to the hormonal system. It's been used for 2000 years and which can make you a genuine Incan warrior during intercourse, therefore the legend tells. Personally, when I have a spoonful of Maca, I get horny just about immediately! And at the top, it has plenty of healing potential too.

Ashwagandha

This one is fantastic too. Started in India, utilized for a large number of years by Ayurvedic practitioners. It's also known as the Indian Ginseng. One study demonstrates *Ashwagandha* stimulates an enzyme referred to as nitric oxide, this can help with the dilating of arteries to the genital organs. It's a brilliant high antioxidant that may increase your libido but also your disease fighting capability.

Cinnamon

Hormone imbalance is normally the root cause with regards to a minimal mojo. Cinnamon is among the popular spices for Christmas but also used since ancient occasions to improve sexual interest.

Yes, you should use one that you currently have within your kitchen or will get to buy nearby. Ideally organic.

Banana

We love bananas. Ok the last one, they have become versatile. Yummy, filled with B vitamins like riboflavin which escalates the body's overall energy. Bananas also contain bromelain enzyme that is believed to support the production of the sex hormones such as testosterone.

Avocado

These likewise have magical strength boosters inside. Avocados contain mineral deposits, monounsaturated fats *(the great kind that protects the heart and lowers cholesterol), and vitamin B6* - all which help to keep your vigor and sex drive up.

Almonds

Selenium might help with infertility issues and, with vitamin E, can help heart health. Zinc is actually a mineral that helps produce men's sex hormones and may boost libido. Blood circulation is very important to your sex organs, so choosing good fats, like the omega-3 fatty acids within almonds, is a genuinely good idea.

Coconut Oil

Without a doubt, this oil is hyped days past, they have incredible sexy use cases, from lubrication to breast massage oil to beautiful skin. Some coconut fanatics say that it could improve your libido, which might be because of antioxidants in the oil that assist combat free radicals that may result in a lowered libido.

Honey

The usage of honey as an aphrodisiac today could be traced back again to many cultures and traditions whereby the sweet sticky liquid is popularly shared between lovers being a sensual food. It is definitely often associated with blissful times, romance, union in marriages, and honeymoon.

Chapter 5

Tips for an Improved Sex Life

Eat Whole-Food Plants

Consuming whole food plants offers you more energy that may lead to improved sex life. A quart of a green smoothie is among the easiest methods for getting 7-10 portions of fruits & vegetables every day.

Among my biggest surprises on paper, the Green Smoothies Diet was discovering that lots of people that drink green smoothies regularly, within my report of 175 people, experience higher libido. (The sex-drive statistic, if you ask me at least, pertains to both vigor and interest in an exceedingly intense, personal reference to other people. In ways, it's just producing your hormones balanced and healthier, and that's an excellent stage too, I believe a higher libido is an all-natural state.) And when plants are everything you eat the majority of, weight loss almost inevitable.

Actually being 10 pounds over your normal weight can vary noticeably affcct libido or trigger low libido. It may seem depressing libido is basically because you don't look sexy or uninhibited when you've got love handles or thigh flab. That's only part of it.

A significant part is a fact that feeling sexy and energetic does result in you being your very self-in in all ways. On the other hand, need to turn the lights off, avoid certain areas of the body being visible, or fretting about insecurities, results in nothing good in the bedroom. The other part is how simply a supplementary 10lbs. truly depresses circulation and endocrine functions. You truly need those functions once and for all lovin'.

Whenever your energy is depleted, since it always is going to be on the typical American Diet diet, you lose the sexual interest and stamina you once had. Sexual dysfunction happens in the same manner all degenerative diseases do: it is linked to lifestyle choices. Your reproductive system, in the end, is suffering from similar things your cardiac, circulatory, and endocrine systems are. All of them are inextricably linked because they are all part of 1 complex organs.

Add these to Your Green;

It's half for you personally and a half for your lover. Here they may be:

Maca

Maca may be the "Peruvian ginseng," a root vegetable prized from the Incans for a large number of years because of its capability to improve athletic endurance and sexual stamina.

Bee pollen

Look what it can for the queen bee! Bee pollen is normally a robust aphrodisiac. Make an effort one grain to be sure you're not allergic and two grains the very next day. Put a spoonful from it within your libido-boosting smoothie when you've ascertained you don't have a sensitivity to it. In addition, it includes a potentially helpful influence on seasonal allergies and immune function! Bee pollen can provide a naturally powerful boost for your libido.

Celery

Yes, the vegetable I affectionately prefer to say originates from the cardboard family. Put it inside your sex smoothie recipe where you won't see it because it contains androsterone, a precursor to pheromones that positively affect the sexual behavior of your lover.

Eat Foods Containing Zinc

Zinc blocks the enzyme that converts testosterone (in charge of libido) into estrogen. Make an effort to also get kidney and lima beans, spinach, some flax, garlic, and peanuts.

Ditch Endocrine-Disrupting Plastics

Don't drink out of plastic containers or microwave stuff in plastic (or, heaven forbid, styrofoam).

Don't Drink Plain Tap Water - Avoid Fluoride and Chlorine

Get yourself a carbon filter overall water system in your house. Get yourself a reverse osmosis filtering, at the very least. On top of that would be to own R.O. water and a water ionizer.

Don't Eat Soy!

Soy and soy-based products have the potential to wreak havoc on your own libido. Most soy inside the U.S. are certainly genetically altered, but worse, processed soy products mimic estrogen in the torso and disrupt the standard hormone function. Don't use soy milk or any other processed soy products; occasionally, smaller amounts of organic miso, edamame, tofu, Nama shoyu, or Bragg's are okay.

Read your labels! You will find soy protein isolate and soy lecithin and twelve other prepared soy fractions in everything boxed, everything canned, and everything manufactured by humans nowadays, including virtually all bread products. Everything accumulates, so cut it out of your daily diet.

Quit Using Chemical-based Skin Products

Make sure the products you utilize on your skin are completely natural to improve your libido. Putting it on your own skin is equivalent to eating it. Your skin layer is a full-time income, breathing organ, and it requires what you placed on it into the bloodstream. Make a shift to the items you placed on your skin layer is only natural. My moisturizer is organic coconut oil.

Review the Drugs You Take

Many over-the-counter and prescription medications suppress libido or causes additional sexual dysfunction. Common culprits are the following:

- ✓ Antihistamines
- ✓ Antidepressants
- ✓ Contraceptive pills or patches
- ✓ Hair thinning treatments
- ✓ Beta-blockers
- ✓ Opioids
- ✓ Medical marijuana

Try turning to a thing that doesn't experience effects on your own libido. Even better, address the primary cause of the problem and that means you can eventually ditch the meds.

Embrace Change of Time

Some people are simply just interested in sex each day, instead of during the night. It's a truism that lots of individuals are either "nighttime people" or "morning people." There's nothing wrong with that. You merely may need to compromise if your lover may be the opposite.

Consult Bioidentical Hormone Specialist

Women obtaining a full blood-panel workup to learn if progesterone or female testosterone may be the base of the problem. Just a little yam-based progesterone or hormone cream may work wonders. (However, you want this only when it's warranted from your test outcomes!) Testosterone cream is suitable only when you are 40 or older.

Please get these only from a bioidentical practitioner. The substances aren't identical to what the body makes. They can be harmful and could involve some symptom-abatement results for a while, but they may also be connected with negative unwanted effects and disease risk. Additional remedies your natural care practitioner may recommend, like DHEA or flax oil, could possibly be very easily located at a health grocery.

Much better than Pills

Each day we are been bombarded with ads recommending male and female medications and herbal treatments for sexual dysfunction. They are actually used in an instant, short-term fix, however, they do not get to solve the main problem, plus they come at a price. Not merely are they expensive, however, they create a growing set of serious unwanted effects such as gastrointestinal problems, memory and vision loss and hearing impairment. Additionally, they hinder the additional medications we take.

So your investment pills! Start juicing for a wholesome and natural enhancement of the sexual experience! Here is a review of the foodstuffs that contain the best concentration of sexually stimulating nutrients - all proven by nutritional research!

Chapter 6

Foods to stay away from

These food types lower libido in men and women, and really should be avoided to be able to ensure the healthy maintenance of your sex life:

Sugar

Processed sugar isn't only unhealthy, it diminishes testosterone in men, thus lowering male libido.

Trans-Fats

Not merely are trans fats nutritionally unhealthy, they lower blood flow and therefore diminish sexual ability in men and women.

Canned Foods

Most cans are lined with *'BPA,'* a substance which, in high levels of exposure have been reported to cause erection dysfunction just as much as four times more regularly in men who consume canned foods frequently. Search for this ***"BPA FREE"*** label on cans.

Soy

Soy lowers libido in men by diminishing testosterone because of the occurrence of estrogen-like compounds.

Salt

Huge amounts of sodium are a source of impotence problems that even medication can not undo.

Alcohol

Though it diminishes inhibition and lessens stress, alcohol lowers our capability to perform and also to get sexually satisfied. Fresh juiced fruits & vegetables with added nuts and spices aren't just a smart way to increase your well-being, strengthen muscle, and reduce weight. Sure combinations, as in the above list, will truly improve your sex life. No matter what your actual age, juicing is among the best methods to have significantly more fun.

Chapter 7

Herbs to Greatly Help with Libido

Maca Root, "Peruvian Viagra"

This funny looking root that originates from the Andes in Peru is making a large splash within the States since it is similar to *Viagra for men and women*. This root will build testosterone in men, and in women, it can help to balance our hormones during menopause while giving us energy and making us feel frisky. This root is classified as an **adaptogen,** and **"Adaptogens"** is a fantastic band of herbs that will help to balance the body. If you want energy, they'll offer you energy, but if you don't sleep, they'll assist you to sleep.

They provide your body what it is missing; you will find about 18 known adaptogens on the planet. When you can add one or a number of these incredible herbs to your food regimen, the healthier you'll be because this reduces your cellular damage due to stress to enable you to age more gracefully and also have fewer wrinkles as you do so. Maca may also assist with infertility, and it accumulates your body's disease fighting capability. This sexy, Peruvian wonder also includes 18 of the fundamental proteins that will be the blocks to protein, so that it can help keep hair and nails healthy, and it can alleviate your symptoms of anxiety and depression. Some women who've had hypothyroidism and started taking Maca could decrease or eliminate their medication after taking it for many months. (I like that! One medicine has gone!). Maca can be filled with Omega-3 oils which help oil up your joints and skin.

Can you envisage having energy, feeling frisky, experiencing no depression or anxiety, and having an excellent hair day?

Now don't you imagine that's sexy? Maca can be purchased in capsules and powder form. You can include the powder to your morning drink or sprinkle it on cereal. It tastes like malt, so this is a quick drink you could ingest in the morning to really get your engine running hot the whole day.

Chocolatemaca shake recipe

Ingredients

- ✓ 2 cups of almond milk

- ✓ 2 spoons of maca powder
- ✓ 1 banana
- ✓ 3-4 cocoa bits
- ✓ Agave syrup to taste

Directions

Blend all ingredients with a few bits of ice and revel in.

Horny Goat Weed, "Yin Yang Huo"

Don't you love the brand of the herb? It is simply totally sexy as well as the brand says it all. It is Viagra within a herb. Horny Goat also supports erection dysfunction and boosts the blood flow to the capillaries and other areas that need blood. It also inhibits estrogen production while increasing your testosterone. If you are a man and you are starting to get a little chubby and feel like you are developing man boobs, it is because you have too much estrogen in your body. When you decrease the estrogen levels, your body will lean out, and the doughy look will disappear.

The cool thing is that there are no side effects when you take this weed, and it won't interfere with your medication. I like the fact that it stimulates both males and females, so you both can feel aroused at the same time and enjoy the sexual fireworks. They have also found that it helps with brain traumas and dementia, so imagine a herb that will help your libido plus you will be able to remember everything on your to-do list.

Horny goat is also a good detoxifier for the liver and kidneys. Could you believe that this sexy herb is the *Trifecta of herbs*? *It helps with your libido, your memory, and also cleanses your liver*.

Pomegranate, "Sexy Ruby Seeds"

Perhaps you have ever seen such beautiful, sexy seeds? They appear to be rubies, and their health advantages are a lot more valuable when compared to a ruby. This antioxidant-rich fruit continues to be revered as symbolic of health, fertility, and eternal life for a long time. These sexy seeds benefit the heart plus the arteries because they increase the speed at which heart blockages melt away. In a study of 84 patients who drank a glass a day, they found that their blood pressure lowered by 12% and plaque by 30%, and those who did not drink the juice saw their plaque levels rise by 9%. Now for the really good news: these crimson beauties can build up your testosterone for both men and women. They help with depression and also help to lower your cholesterol levels. By drinking a glass a day, you can help lower your cholesterol, protect your skin with some potent antioxidants, and it will keep you feeling turned on and sexy all day long.

Antioxidant-rich smoothie

Ingredients:

- ✓ 4 cups of baby spinach
- ✓ ½ cup of pomegranate juice
- ✓ ½ cup of blueberries frozen
- ✓ ½ cup of strawberries frozen
- ✓ 4 dates, cut in two
- ✓ 1 tablespoon of flaxseed,
- ✓ ground ½ avocado,

Instruction:

Blend all of the ingredients together and revel in.

L-Dopa Mucuna, "The Sexy Velvet Bean"

These ebony color beans have become sexy due to the beautiful things they can do to help your brain and body greatly. **L-dopa** can be any amino acid that the body needs to produce *Dopamine* for the human brain. The neurotransmitter Dopamine is in charge of providing you that fantastic feeling of pleasure. In the event that you feel like you will have a cloud over your mind and cannot appear to shake it, you then should consider taking *Dopa Mucuna* because your dopamine levels may be low.

It will also help you to sleep, and it stops the nightly chatter in your head before bed so you can go right to sleep. In India and Brazil, Dopa-Mucuna is known as a powerful aphrodisiac because it helps build up testosterone in the body. It also builds up the Human Growth Hormone (HGH) in your body, so you get two powerful hormones to help stimulate your libido and give you a sense of joy. When you ingest the *Dopa Mucona*, the body can assimilate the HGH and use it: yet, if you take HGH in capsules it can cause inflammation because it has been forced into the body, and the body doesn't know how to use it. Imagine feeling friskier, joyful, and getting a really good night's rest. Your sleep will improve, and your mood will improve exponentially because the *L-dopa* takes away the cloud and improves your sleep.

It also calms your nervous system and balances out all your hormones. L-Dopa Mucona can be purchased in pill form or powder form, and some muscle powders are adding it to their mixes as well. I would recommend taking 1-2 capsules a day to keep those ugly clouds away, so you can feel sexy and sunny every day. If you are having a problem with depression along with the black clouds, you might want to add 5HTP (which helps build up your serotonin levels) with the L-dopa so that you can balance out two neurotransmitters instead of one and really see the sun breaking through the clouds. One way to tell if your dopamine levels are low is if you crave sugar. Sugar burns up your dopamine, so if you eat a lot of refined carbohydrates, you will start losing your natural joy. Sugar gives you a temporary feeling of joy, but it is definitely short-lived, and then it makes the problem worse, so you will crave more hope that you will feel well again. I recommend taking L-dopa to stop the craving for sugar and then trying to look for things in your life that offer you sweetness and delight instead of looking for a sense of sweetness in your daily life exclusively from your food intake.

Yohimbre Bark, "The Super Viagra"

This incredibly sexy bark that originates from the Congo region of Africa possesses some very exciting properties. This bark might help with erection dysfunction as various other herbs can, but what's ground-breaking is the fact in addition, it helps with erection dysfunction that's worsened or due to taking antidepressants, heart pressure medicine, or from being diabetic. Many of these medications make it very hard for herbs to greatly help with erection dysfunction, but that one does not hinder the medication. It bypasses the medication and increases blood circulation just to the groin region.

How exciting is that? This herb also has the ability to help women who have lost their desire for sex because of their antidepressants or other medications that they are taking.

Women don't have to worry about obtaining it up, but if our hearts and minds are not in it, we might as well call it a day because we won't get excited. This herb helps you to get aroused while it gets your mind and body to get in sync, so all you have to do is kick back and enjoy the ride. *How is this incredible bark able to help people with diabetes and people on high blood pressure medicine?*

It works because it contains a chemical called ***"yohimbine,"*** which can increase blood flow and nerve impulses to the penis or vagina. This increases desire and stamina without interfering with medication or elevating the heart rate. I am very excited about this herb because I have tried to help patients with erectile dysfunction who are taking these medications, and the results were not that great until recently.

This bark can also help with weight loss and energy. Weightlifters use it to improve their workout performances. I know it seems like this is a miracle herb, but I would really like to emphasize the benefits for people who have erectile dysfunction and how exciting it is to get your desire back for both men and women. Many people taking anti-depressants just chalk it up to, "oh well, I guess

I will have to deal with low libido, but at least I am not so depressed and irritable all the time." Now with Yohimbe, you can be calm, cool, and collected while still enjoying wonderful sex life. Now, don't you think that is something to cheer about? This sexy bark can be purchased online, and many health food stores in tincture, powders, and tablets. Take the Yohimbe daily to clear out the blood vessels and build up desire and stamina.

Saw Palmetto Berries

These sexy berries will keep your man's prostate healthy and keep him virile for a long period. A lot of men experience benign prostatic hyperplasia (BPH) if they start to get older that is due to their prostates swelling up. BPH can result in an array of symptoms like increased urinary frequency, a weak urination stream, and difficulty initiating urination. Saw Palmetto would help with these symptoms, and in lots of countries like Germany, Italy, and Austria, this herb may be the first type of defence against BPH. Within the united states, men often prescribed Flomax to help significantly using their symptoms, plus some of the yucky unwanted effects of taking Flomax are a dry mouth, abnormal ejaculation, dizziness, runny nose, and a sore back. Saw Palmetto, on the other hand, has no known side effects.

Saw Palmetto can also raise testosterone, which will cause a higher libido. It will also reduce hair loss, and it helps to build muscle tissue because it is so high in essential fatty acids that bind to the protein molecules to build muscle mass. Imagine a husband who is suffering from an enlarged prostate, a runny nose, dry throat, sore back, and dizziness. Now imagine a husband who has an enlarged prostate that is getting smaller, his hair is growing in, his muscles are becoming more defined, and his libido is up. How I just love herbs, and I think that they are so sexy compared to Western medications.

Cnidium Monnier, "Natural Libido Booster"

This herb has been used for a large number of years in Traditional Chinese Medicine as an aphrodisiac and a libido booster. It can support the body to create nitric oxide, which helps your body to mail blood for the penis, which means you can feature stronger and more durable erections. If your trouble is early ejaculation, this herb will help you prolong your erection for a bit longer. Cnidium

Monnier is yellow seeds that come through the same family as the carrot and fennel.

These sexy seeds may also support women because they can send blood in your clitoris such that it engorges, and it becomes very sensitive. You should have some terrific orgasms, and these sexy seeds will put you in the mood for increasingly more. Another delightful effect of taking Cnidium is the fact that it can help with vaginal dryness, and as the clitoris feels so sensitive, it can benefit from frigidity too. This libido enhancer also really helps to strengthen your bones, and it is a warming tonic for your body so that it also offers a gentle strengthening influence on the complete body. These sexy seeds promote vigor and present the body a good sense of wellbeing and can hopefully put a laugh on your own face.

Damiana, "Mayan Sexual Enhancer"

This herb grows in Mexico and Texas and continues to be used because the *Mayans* have already been gazing on the stars and developing their incredible calendar. They may have used it as an aphrodisiac and a sexual rejuvenator for men who experience impotence. What I love about *Damiana* is that it's an over-all tonic for your body, so it might help with exhaustion and overall weakness. *Damiana* can build-up your energy and strength, and hopefully, you then will begin to desire intimacy. It really is hard to want sex if you are merely completely exhausted and weak on a regular basis. This sexy herb may also help relax your nervous system and help with depression and anxiety. They have also found it very useful for those who have problems with the obsessive compulsive disorder (OCD) since it might help calm the racing mind and settle anxiousness.

This sexy Mayan secret may also regulate the number of female hormones in the torso, so it might help with menopause and hot flashes. Imagine not being exhausted, feeling happy, or content, rather than having hot flashes; now doesn't that make you feel just a little friskier? This herb could be used alone or together with similar herbs to create it better. They state it is effective will Saw Palmetto that helps the prostate, and for a few men, it gave them a mild sense of euphoria. I believe a euphoric feeling in the bedroom before anything happens could be pretty exciting.

Tribulus Terrestries, "Muscle Builder and Sexual Enhancer All in a Single"

This herb may also be called *"Puncture vine,"* and it's been used for years and years in Asia and in Eastern Europe. In Asia, it's been used as a libido enhancer in both men and women since it helps to increase testosterone in the torso. Tribulus produces a steroid called *"protodioscin"* that converts androgen into testosterone or estrogen, whichever your body needs so that it helps balance the hormones. This sexy vine also produces **DHEA,** which may be the precursor for all your hormones in the torso; therefore, it makes sure that your testosterone keeps on being made by the body.

In case your testosterone is low, it could improve the testosterone to a standard level, and it could hold it there for a long time. The reason why I said for some time is that I want you to definitely choose Tribulus for 2-3 months each day and then quit for a month and then return back again. In the event that you set it off for some time, it lets your body understand that it can't rest on its laurels and must keep on producing testosterone. Your body will continue vacation and prevent carrying out its work if you continue giving your body what it is missing. We wish the body to start working again rather than continually be counting on herbs, creams, or pills. We just desire to provide it with a loving push to get started again. Lots of the herbal formulas which they sell have Tribulus in it, which is an essential thing. I do like it blended with different herbs and not simply alone to provide it with a larger punch. The dosage is 85-250mg, three times per day, for three months, and off for a month, and then back for another three months.

Ginkgo Biloba, "Medicinal Leaves From The Oldest Living Tree Species"

The Ginkgo Biloba tree 's been around for over 15-20 million years, and its leaves have already been found in Chinese as medicine for a large number of years. The leaves are recognized to assist with circulation, also to obtain oxygen and nutrients to all of the body and to promote longevity. There were many reports done on what it can benefit from memory and cognitive abilities; however, they are also researching what it can help with having blood right down to the male sex organ and exactly how it can benefit with infertility and erection dysfunction.

Can you envisage how wonderful it might be to reside with a guy in whom both of his heads will work at an optimal level? You can begin moaning, saying that he never forgets how exactly to please you because he's a Ginkgo Biloba man!" This 'oldie but goodie' herb may also aid in asthma, allergies, and it could relax the lungs if they are in circumstances of inflammation since it delivers pure oxygen to the lungs. Additionally, it may improve peripheral vascular disease, and it breaks up platelets and helps the blood to flow more freely.

Please, do not consider it if you're on the blood thinner or are inclined to seizures but also for ordinary people should take at least 40-80 milligrams, three times every day, so as to be sharp and alert on a regular basis.

www.ingramcontent.com/pod-product-compliance
Lightning Source LLC
Chambersburg PA
CBHW071514210326
41597CB00018B/2755